THE PATIENT'S HEALTHCARE ADVOCATE

THE PATIENT'S HEALTHCARE ADVOCATE

PROFESSIONAL TIPS AND EXPERT ADVICE ON HOW TO MAXIMIZE INSURANCE BENEFITS AND REDUCE COSTS

JOHN MOYLE

The Patient's Healthcare Advocate

Cover Art: Jennifer Toomey

ISBN: 978-1-7332443-0-5

The views, opinions, recommendations, and information communicated in this text are provided solely by the author, drawing from his personal and professional experience, and do not necessarily reflect the policies, positions, instructions, thoughts, or opinions of any insurance agency, medical provider, patient, pharmaceutical company, medical company, or employer in any form or fashion.

This information is meant to support all aspects of the healthcare system by describing possible perspectives of each entities' viewpoint. My hope is to cultivate improved health outcomes, by doing what I believe to be ethically and morally upstanding, through transparent patient advocacy and education. By natural extension, I also see it as a way of supporting health insurance companies and medical providers both, who also need patients to understand their policies and systems of communication. Patients will develop a trusting and loyal relationship when they have a better understanding of how each process works, realistic expectations, and a reduction in unexpected bills.

The material listed in this book is from my own phrasing, is common knowledge across the health insurance industry, is common knowledge throughout most of the medical field, and is all available to insurance consumers through one means or another. The book simply condenses the information into an easily understood quick-reference guide. All information written in this text was information that I was allowed to tell clients, members, and patients. None of it was restricted information that a patient, member, or client was not privy to. Although, the information is based on a healthcare worker's perspective, none of it is a disclosure of internal secrets or other information restricted to any specific company, internal communication only, or an organization's employees only.

None of the information listed in this book, was forbidden for me to tell a client of the insurance company or a patient when helping them resolve insurance related issues. Each topic has been something I've experienced in the past, as a patient continuously facing problems with my medical insurance, care coordination, and claims. I've personally experienced, assisted a friend, assisted a family member, assisted a patient, and assisted an insurance client with each of these scenarios in some form or another. I've been involved in each topic, from at least two different perspectives, depending on the case. There have been times when I've had to call the insurance to have medical services covered, because I was given incorrect information, as a patient and on behalf of a patient while working as a nurse practitioner.

Although the text primarily refers to preferred provider plans, also known as PPO health insurance plans, the principles described in the text can easily apply towards many other forms of medical and prescription insurance.

CONTENTS

INTRODUCTION

Have you experienced intense frustration and confusion when dealing with your health insurance company? Welcome to the club! Far too many of us are familiar with the distress of rejected prescriptions, denied or delayed medical services, and unexpected medical bills.

For countless people, dealing with the modern healthcare system is a singular hell. Many patients feel that they're paying more every year for premiums but receiving less coverage. Never before has navigating one's healthcare been so difficult. High deductibles, large out-of-pocket costs, prior authorizations, plan exclusions, and ever-shrinking benefits have led to a generally negative view of health insurance companies.

Doctors can write prescriptions and order diagnostic tests all day long, but too often patients find themselves unable to access them—due to costs, misunderstandings, and other barriers. Faced with such obstacles, patients often give up and go without medical care instead of looking into additional resources. This places their health at risk and causes them to think of their insurance as the enemy. Sure, you can complain about the healthcare system and hope for large-scale reform (and I wouldn't blame you), but is that going to help you in your moment of need?

You might assume that, since you're paying your premiums for insurance coverage, the doctor's office and the insurance company should be working together to streamline your care. Sadly, that's not how the system works. The burden of responsibility falls on you, the patient, to coordinate care for yourself.

Yes, to ensure a smooth process in receiving benefits, it's the *patient's responsibility* to coordinate with every party involved and make sure nothing has been missed. The patient must proactively make sure the doctor's office, the pharmacy, the medical supply company, the medical facility, and the health insurance company are all on the same page.

If that sounds like a tall order, here's the good news: I've written this book to streamline the healthcare process as much as possible for you. It is fundamental that patients know how their insurance plans work and how to effectively utilize their benefits. Unfortunately, the complexity of coordinating your healthcare, often leads to an array of problems. Thanks to my many years of working in the healthcare industry—as a registered nurse at a large hospital, as a nurse practitioner in the nonprofit sector, and as a customer care advocate for a major health insurance agency—combined with my experiences as a patient in need of medical benefits—I offer a very unique insider's perspective.

With this book, my goal is to empower patients, by explaining how health insurance works and outlining which steps to take to coordinate care and avoid costly mistakes. In this guide, you will find the information you need to make purposeful, educated choices, enjoy benefits, and avoid the most common pitfalls of insurance plan holders today. You will discover that there are cost-effective options when dealing with the doctor's office, the pharmacy, the hospital, and imaging facilities.

I've structured this book around the most common complaints and questions that I have heard as an insurance customer care advocate. In each case, I will set realistic expectations in a section called "Reality Check"; provide information that I've learned from professional and personal experiences under "Healthcare Knowledge"; and lay out clear steps you can take to advocate for yourself under "Responsible Research."

At the end, I've compiled a Patient's Checklist, a concise list of all the most vital information. The Healthcare Checklist helps you effectively navigate the complex world of health insurance by listing the most practical tips and takeaways for preventing problems and unexpected expenses, followed by a Frequently Asked Questions section to address more specific concerns. For your convenience, I've also provided a glossary of common terms that appear throughout the book. Feel free to jump around to the sections that are most relevant to you at any given time, and keep the book handy as an ongoing reference.

Armed with all of the knowledge in this guide, you will be able to navigate the healthcare system with far greater ease, advocate for your own healthcare needs, and claim the benefits to which you are entitled. When faced with healthcare obstacles, you must persevere, and conquer them!

CHAPTER 1

HOW MODERN HEALTH INSURANCE WORKS

"Isn't it up to the doctor's office and my insurance to make sure I'm getting billed correctly?"

Like many people, you might believe that your insurance company is the link holding all the pieces of your healthcare together, but it's actually you, the patient, at the center of it all. You are the raison d'être for the insurance company, the medical providers, the service facilities, and pharmacies. They all exist to serve you, and they all depend on you to coordinate them. It is up to you to ensure that they are communicating with one another and processing the claims correctly.

Health plans work by shielding you from the high costs of medical care. You pay a monthly premium to maintain health insurance coverage. In order to benefit from these coverages, most plans require that you meet a deductible before the insurance benefits actually apply. Once you meet the deductible, the health insurance plan covers a portion of your healthcare expenses. If you utilize an in-network provider, facility, or pharmacy, you benefit from the contracted rate.

REALITY CHECK: ONE TYPE OF INSURANCE DOESN'T COVER EVERYTHING

Your health insurance covers your medical needs; your prescription insurance covers your medication needs; your dental insurance covers your dental needs; and your vision insurance covers your eye care, prescription glasses, and contact lenses. Each of these insurance companies usually has its own vendor company who manages the plan. Except in rare cases, these four basic categories of health care—medical, prescription medication, dental, and vision—are commonly covered by separate insurance companies and vendors.

However, some health insurance plans do cover a combination of these categories. When this happens, each category is handled by separate departments within the insurance company, even in the rare cases that they are handled by the same vendor.

HEALTHCARE KNOWLEDGE: WHO CHOOSES WHAT'S COVERED IN YOUR PLAN?

Contrary to popular belief, the insurance company does not choose your coverages, exclusions, or medication list. The insurance company provides your employer with all of the possible options and the employer picks and chooses what they can afford and will cover for their employees. (If you are self-employed, then you choose these items for yourself.)

RESPONSIBLE RESEARCH: PERSONAL NEEDS DICTATE WHICH TYPE OF PLAN FITS YOU BEST

Each health insurance plan is different, and it's important to be aware of your options. There are plans with high deductibles and low premiums, plans with low deductibles and high premiums, and plans that are a mix of both. People who require a high amount of medical care would probably benefit from a plan with a high premium and a low deductible that has a large network of medical providers. Very healthy people who rarely use their medical coverage may benefit from a high-deductible, low-premium plan. However, I have seen people with this latter type of plan face huge costs due to unexpected surgeries, pregnancies, and major health changes. I recommend that you protect yourself by choosing a low-deductible plan unless you have the funds to cover a high-deductible one at your disposal.

Additionally, there are plans that have a great number of medical providers and others that are restricted to a select few providers in that region. Depending on the area in which you live, you may prefer one type of plan over the other. In general, however, I recommend that you choose the plan type that has a wide range of medical providers, as this eliminates the risk of having to wait for an extended period of time or having to drive to other cities to see a clinician in your network.

CHAPTER 2

UNEXPECTED BILLS

"Oh, I just have a really quick question. Once I meet my deductible, everything is covered at 100 percent, right?"

REALITY CHECK: READ YOUR BENEFIT PACKAGE

It's important that you know the details specific to your insurance plan. At minimum, you should be aware of your deductible, copays, co-insurances, and prescription coverage details. When you choose a plan during open enrollment, make sure you read the benefit package details. (If you're the spouse or dependent of the primary insurance subscriber, ask them for details about the benefits or create an account online with your social security number and birth date to access information about your benefits.) Granted, reading your benefit package is not the most exciting thing to do, but it is necessary if you want to avoid all kinds of headaches and unexpected bills in the coming year. Your future self will thank you for it!

RESPONSIBLE RESEARCH: CPT CODES

Current Procedural Technology codes, commonly known as CPT codes, are important billing codes for patients to be aware of, as they determine what benefit will cover the charges. CPT codes are what the doctor will use to bill for the services they provide. Every time a doctor orders blood work, imaging, procedures, diagnostic testing, or schedules a surgery, ask the doctor's office for the CPT code they'll use for billing. Then call the insurance company and ask them to check the CPT code to determine which benefit the procedure falls under, if it is a covered health service that is considered medically necessary. The insurance company cannot generate CPT codes for you based on any other information you provide. In order to present you with accurate information, they must have the CPT codes from the medical provider. The CPT codes will allow the insurance agent to determine if it's covered under your plan as well as alert the agent to tell you if the procedure has certain requirements for coverage or if prior authorization is necessary. Having the relevant CPT codes ready when you call your health insurance company will save you time and frustration.

SELF-ADVOCACY: IN-NETWORK V. OUT-OF-NETWORK

To make your insurance plan work for you, it's essential to determine *before* you see a medical provider whether that provider is in-network. An in-network provider or facility is one that has contracted with your health insurance company to accept certain negotiated rates, which are usually significantly lower than those offered by out-of-network providers.

The next step is to investigate how the provider bills for their services. Sometimes they may bill under their name; other times under the facility's name. Find this out to determine if they are in-network or not.

In certain circumstances, it may be difficult to find an in-network provider, but it is necessary to avoid unexpected expenses. For example, when a patient is admitted to an in-network hospital and seen by a hospitalist during their stay, the hospitalist is not guaranteed to be in-network. A hospitalist is commonly known as a doctor who cares for patients while they're hospitalized. Understandably, patients tend to assume that hospitalists are covered at the in-network benefit—but this is not always the case.

Generally speaking, medical providers seen at an in-network facility are covered at the in-network rate. This rule most often applies when a patient is seen by an anesthesiologist, radiologist, or pathologist at an in-network facility. Hospitalists, however, are notorious for being out of network while seeing patients during their hospital stay. They are less likely to be covered at the in-network rate and aren't usually covered by the same benefit clause as anesthesiologists, pathologists, and radiologists are.

With very few exceptions, a patient has the right to refuse medical service. You can decline services from a medical provider who isn't participating in your plan, and try to find one who is, to avoid out-of-network bills. However, if you turn away a hospitalist, there may not be another in-network hospitalist available. This is one of those distressing predicaments for which there's no easy solution, but you *can* advocate for yourself in an effort to find an answer. During my time as an insurance customer care advocate, I have found this to be a common source of frustration for patients who have sought my assistance. It seems that the only thing a patient can do is ask a nurse manager to help them find another hospitalist to see them, and check if the other hospitalists available are in their network, or address the bill after they've been discharged from the hospital.

Despite all of these variables, your health and safety are the main priority. None of the above is a justification to forego medical care. In other words, *do not ever go without health services if you think you need them.* Just remember that when a provider is assigned to you by the hospital, you can look into their network status and seek a provider who is participating in your plan. If an out-of-network provider treats you in the hospital, you can attempt to address the issue while in the hospital, or appeal the bill afterward if it's not covered at the in-network rate. In any case, do not ever compromise or risk your health by going without care.

HEALTHCARE KNOWLEDGE: A POSSIBLE LOOPHOLE FOR UNEXPECTED OUT-OF-NETWORK HOSPITALIST OR ER PHYSICIAN BILLS

If you're charged an out-of-network rate for an out-of-network hospitalist or emergency room doctor who saw you while you were at an in-network hospital, you should appeal the charge. A general rule of thumb in health insurance is "the place of service drives the benefit." In other words, the best way to appeal this charge is by finding language in your benefit package, with verbiage that supports why the out-of-network hospitalist's fees should be covered at the in-network benefit. Look for language along the lines of the following: inpatient benefits cover services received during the hospital stay and physician services. Services include those performed by consulting medical providers or emergency room doctors.

Specific language about "consulting" or "emergency room" medical providers, listed directly in your benefit coverages, could be your saving grace. You can argue that it's clearly stated that your in-network inpatient hospital stay benefits cover "services by consulting physicians." Since the consulting physician saw you while you were an inpatient at an in-network hospital, you should be covered at the in-network rate. They may still find a way to deny the claim, but this is the only loophole I've been able to find regarding coverage for out-of-network hospitalist bills.

ON A PERSONAL NOTE

It's my personal belief that hospitalists should be covered by the in-network hospital-inpatient stay benefit as the other medical providers are. It's nearly impossible to choose your hospitalists, so why are they not covered at the in-network rate like anesthesiologists, radiologists, and pathologists are when you receive care from an in-network hospital? I genuinely don't know why this is the case. Fixing this incongruity necessitates ongoing healthcare reform. In the absence of such clauses, patients must be aware of this issue and the options available to them as outlined above.

CHAPTER 3

LAB WORK

"Why did I receive a bill for eight hundred dollars on blood work? I went to where my doctor told me to go to get my blood drawn in his office! Now you are making me choose between feeding my kids and paying this bill! Why wasn't it covered?"

REALITY CHECK: DOCTORS ORDER LAB WORK BASED ON NEED, NOT COVERAGE

Doctors choose lab work based on medical, not health insurance coverage. When ordering your bloodwork, the doctor is thinking about your health and does not know the cost of the labs. Their decisions are based on your medical care, not the details related to your health insurance. The test that your doctor is recommending for you may not be covered by your plan, may be costly, or may require prior authorization to prove that it is medically necessary.

HEALTHCARE KNOWLEDGE: CONVENIENCE V. COVERAGE

Doctors order lab work based on your personalized medical needs, while they recommend lab facilities based on convenience and location, but it is your responsibility to determine whether the lab company is in-network or not. Most doctors' offices have an onsite lab station, but the phlebotomist is usually working for a third-party lab company, not for the doctor's office. Most patients assume that the phlebotomist is employed by the doctor's office and don't think to ask which lab their blood work will be sent to, which makes it easy to see why this problem occurs.

When a doctor says, "Go get your labs drawn," the patient might understandably assume that the lab company is in-network. This is not always the case. Your insurance company may not be in-network with the company that the phlebotomist works for and sends your blood work to. This is a very common issue and patients are frequently caught off guard, so be sure that lab company is in-network before you get your blood drawn.

RESPONSIBLE RESEARCH: ASK ABOUT THE LAB COMPANY

Ask your doctor for the name of the lab company that works with their office. Once you find that out, determine if that lab company is in-network. If it's out-of-network, ask your doctor for an order form for a lab that's in-network. This takes extra time and effort but will save you a considerable amount of frustration and unnecessary cost later. You can then take the order form to one of the lab company's offices to have your blood drawn. Doctors won't know if the lab company working in their office is in your network, so you must determine this for yourself.

As an extra precaution, when you see the phlebotomist, ask them which lab company they are sending your labs to, and tell them what lab facility is in-network with you—so that you, the clinician, and the phlebotomist are all on the same page.

CHAPTER 4

DIAGNOSTIC TESTING

"Why isn't the test covered at 100 percent? What is the point of paying health insurance premiums if you have to meet a deductible? I can't afford to pay $1,000 for this MRI!"

REALITY CHECK: DOCTORS ORDER DIAGNOSTICS BASED ON NEED, NOT COVERAGE

Doctors choose diagnostic imaging based on medical need, not a patient's benefits. Just like lab work, a diagnostic test may not be covered or may require prior authorization to ensure it is medically necessary, safe, and effective. Again, the doctor is thinking about your health, not your coverage, and will not know the cost of the diagnostic imaging.

HEALTHCARE KNOWLEDGE: EACH TESTING FACILITY OFFERS DIFFERENT RATES

Doctors choose imaging facilities based on convenience, location, and their charting system. The doctor is not thinking about the cost of one place versus another. Large hospitals charge more than freestanding facilities do, for the same exact diagnostic test. For example, a large hospital may charge $1,000 for an MRI of the lumbar spine, while a freestanding facility may only charge $300 for the same test.

RESPONSIBLE RESEARCH: FIND A FACILITY THAT CHARGES LESS

Ask your doctor for the CPT code and the exact name of the diagnostic test. Once you have this information, you can begin searching for the in-network facility that charges the least for the same test. You can call the insurance benefits department to have a customer service rep help you. They'll assist you by providing a list of facilities with the lowest out-of-pocket cost for the test the doctor ordered. Most customer service reps have access to a program, where they can enter the name of the imaging or diagnostic test the doctor ordered, that will generate a list of facilities near you with the lowest cost. This could save you thousands of dollars each year. Once you've determined which facility to use, tell your doctor's office where to send the imaging order. As long as there are no specific reasons the doctor requires you to go to a specific facility, the office should comply.

FURTHER FINANCIAL ASSISTANCE MAY BE AVAILABLE

If the least expensive facility is still too expensive for your budget, ask the imaging facility if they have a financial assistance program or if they offer any form of patient assistance. Even if you've met your deductible, a "major diagnostic" test such as an MRI or CT scan can still be highly expensive. Patients delay or go without medical imaging for many reasons, such as being uninsured, having a very limited income, and/or having chosen a high-deductible medical insurance plan. When these situations arise, ask the imaging facility about patient assistance programs to help cover out-of-pocket costs.

Remember, there is some form of assistance for most types of medical care, but you must actively look for it. It comes in many forms. Hospitals often have "financial counselors" that can go over assistance options with you. Do not give up!

ON A PERSONAL NOTE

Ask the imaging facility if they have any form of patient assistance program. I was unaware that any imaging facility would have a patient assistance program until recently, when I had to have several tests done myself. After learning of this resource, I was able to help uninsured patients obtain diagnostic testing and help patients with high-deductible plans afford their imaging tests.

Not all imaging facilities have patient assistance programs, but it is worth the time and effort to inquire about these type of programs, especially if you're in a financial bind. This is another example of why it is so important to look into other resources before giving up on addressing your healthcare needs.

CHAPTER 5

AT THE DOCTOR'S OFFICE

"My doctor was in my network for the past ten years with my previous insurance. Why am I getting a bill saying that he is out of network?"

REALITY CHECK: CONSENTS AND RESPONSIBILITY FOR CHARGES

Signing consents, contracts, and patient paperwork is a necessary evil if you want to be seen by a doctor for medical care. By doing so, you're accepting responsibility for the charges—whatever they may be. It's the patient's responsibility to verify if the doctor, address, and facility are in-network. Every plan is different and changes are made to most plans every year, so check the status before each medical appointment.

HEALTHCARE KNOWLEDGE: A CAUTIONARY TALE

The front desk staff at the doctor's office generally try to be efficient and helpful, but they are only human, and given the sheer volume of patients and paperwork flowing in and out of the office each day, you can see why unintentional mistakes often occur. Although formal medical receptionist programs are available, many of these staff members only receive a few weeks of on-the-job training.

Front desk staff are often overworked and underappreciated. Many times, in my own experience as a patient, they have accidentally pulled up the wrong plan when verifying my medical insurance benefits. If something sounds odd or incorrect, kindly ask them to try again and link your current insurance with your visit. If you know that the information they've told you is inconsistent with what you know to be true about your benefits, respectfully request that they recheck their system and reverify your benefits. If you receive a lot of push-back, it's best to avoid a negative interaction and simply ask another receptionist to help you resolve the issue."

Last year, I went to a doctor's office for a sick visit. At the time, I knew that I had met my in-network deductible and out-of-pocket maximum for the calendar year. The first red flag popped up when the front desk employee told me that the insurance they verified was showing a different ID number than the card I had on me, which I knew was the card connected to my current coverage. I was so sick that I didn't think anything of this and was seen by my doctor. Afterward, when I was checking out, I was told I owed $137 for this office visit.

Since I knew I had met my out-of-pocket costs for the year and the two receptionists would not admit the error, I had to get the office manager involved. The office manager did as I asked, and rechecked the system to verify my benefits. I was correct: The receptionist had found an old plan that was clearly marked terminated and showed that I had not met my deductible. That plan was more than six years old and from a previous employer. If I had not advocated for myself, I would've been overcharged and faced with the frustration of trying to obtain a refund from them after the fact. This type of error happens on a daily basis at doctors' offices across the nation, but most people don't know that they're being wrongfully charged. Advocate for yourself and don't let this happen to you.

RESPONSIBLE RESEARCH: CHECK YOUR MEDICAL PROVIDER'S NETWORK STATUS

Every time you change jobs, obtain a new health insurance plan, renew during open enrollment, or switch to a different plan within the same company, check to see if the provider and facility you use will be in-network. A directory of in-network providers that accept your type of plan may not be available until after you're in the new plan, which can be frustrating, but if possible it's better to know sooner rather than later so you can find an in-network provider and location before the new plan takes effect.

Keep in mind that if a doctor's office says they accept your type of insurance, it doesn't necessarily mean they're in-network with your type of plan. Sometimes a doctor can be in-network but the location is new and there's not yet an in-network contract for that location.

Each year, once your new insurance cycle begins, you have the opportunity to check to make sure your provider and facility are in-network. The doctor may have changed what type of insurance plans they'll accept for that new year, or your plan may have changed which medical providers are in-network for the new year. The bottom line is you need to verify that both the medical provider and the location of service are in-network with your plan, when the new plan begins.

SELF-ADVOCACY: ASK YOUR DOCTOR'S OFFICE TO SUBMIT A PRE-D

A pre-D, or predetermination of benefits, is advantageous for circumventing insurance-related issues and unexpected costs. A pre-D is a letter of request that the doctor's office submits to the insurance company to assess coverage and responsibility of costs. More specifically, the pre-D is submitted to the insurance's clinical service department to examine the billing codes, diagnosis codes, and medical information. In turn, the clinical service department sends the estimate of coverage and responsibility of costs back to your doctor's office. In turn, someone from the doctor's office will usually call to notify you of the estimate. However, if you don't hear back within a reasonable amount of time, follow up with them to make sure nothing has fallen through the cracks. This process does take time—up to two weeks—but it can save you thousands of dollars in the long run by preemptively catching errors.

To prevent unexpected bills, request that your doctor's office submit a pre-D for every service they order, so that you'll have a realistic estimate of your expected costs. Remember, doctors don't know your coverage, so it's up to you to advocate on your behalf to get this information.

CHAPTER 6

THE PRE-APPROVAL PROCESS

"Why do I have to wait for an approval for a surgery that my doctor told me I need? Why hasn't it been approved yet? My surgery is scheduled for tomorrow!"

REALITY CHECK: A PRE-APPROVAL REQUIRES MULTIPLE STEPS

Pre-approval is commonly known as a prior authorization or PA. Doctor's submit PA requests to insurance companies to obtain pre-approval for certain medications, diagnostic tests, and procedures. Most pre-approvals take a minimum of five to fifteen days to process. Each doctor's order and/or prescription goes through several steps of processing, and each step can take days to complete. A doctor will order medication, imaging, or a procedure based on your medical needs without knowing if this will need a prior authorization or not. Once they submit the order and prescription, they may be alerted a day or two later if it needs a PA. That PA will then go on the doctor's list of paperwork to complete and submit for clinical review. The insurance company will review it to make sure the medication, procedure, and/or imaging ordered by the doctor is consistent with current medical guidelines that are proven to be safe and effective for the patient's diagnosis.

A prior authorization occurs when your doctor requests pre-approval for specific medical services. The medical provider's goal is to submit patient-specific documentation that proves the service is medically necessary. When a medical provider requests prior authorization, they're submitting your clinical information and stating why the medical service needs to be completed for your specific diagnosis. Often, you must have proof that you've tried basic treatments for your disorder that have not yielded any improvement. A prior authorization is both a request for the service and the actual decision made by the insurance company. The insurance company may approve or deny pre-approval, or request additional documentation before making a decision.

If your prior authorization is denied because you did not meet the very specific criteria that determine if the service is medically necessary or not, you still have some options. If your healthcare provider still believes you need the service, after they've reviewed why your pre-approval was denied, they can often call a medical director in the prior-authorization department to plead your case. If the medical director agrees with your medical provider, they can override the decision and have the service approved. If this option is not available, your provider can always submit an appeal to fight the decision. If the provider thinks this decision was reached in error, they can submit an appeal, stating why your medical condition requires the service.

HEALTHCARE KNOWLEDGE: WHY PAs ARE NECESSARY AND TIME-CONSUMING

Generally, patients feel frustrated with the pre-approval process. As a customer care advocate, I've heard hundreds of complaints from patients that they feel they shouldn't have to go through a PA for this test or that procedure. After all, their doctor ordered it, so it's what they need for their condition—why should the insurance company need to review it?

Disappointingly, some doctors have been known to order excessive, unnecessary, and/or unsafe treatments that didn't meet medical standards. Because of the history of abuse within the system, insurance companies now pick through each request with a fine-tooth comb. It's unfortunate that the process is so extensive and cumbersome, but it is now required to ensure the treatment procedure is safe, medically effective, cost effective, and adheres to current guidelines.

Every day, a patient will call me to complain, "My doctor told me you still haven't approved my surgery yet. What's the holdup? Are you trying to kill me?" Invariably, when I go to check the status of the PA, I see that the doctor's office only just faxed in the medical documentation and clinical information one or two days before, for a surgery that's just one or two days away. The doctor's office has told the patient that the insurance hasn't approved the surgery yet, but they neglected to tell the patient that they only recently submitted the PA paperwork.

A PA can take two to fifteen days for a variety of reasons, depending on whether is it urgent or standard, whether more medical documentation is needed, and whether the medical documentation was incomplete—combined with the time it takes for a registered nurse and/or medical director to review it.

RESPONSIBLE RESEARCH: START THE PROCESS ASAP AND FOLLOW UP

Initiate the PA process early for any medication, imaging, or procedure that your doctor orders. If you know you're going to have a procedure, make sure to ask your doctor's office to submit the pre-approval on time—two to three weeks *before* the scheduled date of the procedure. If any gaps need to be closed or bumps in the road need to be smoothed out along the way, you and your doctor's office will have time to address any issues well in advance. This will spare you a great deal of stress and frustration.

CHAPTER 7

PRESCRIPTIONS

"Are you are trying to kill me? You denied my medication! I've been on it for five years and nothing else works. Why was it denied? What are you going to do to fix this?"

REALITY CHECK: YOUR MEDICAL PLAN IS NOT YOUR PRESCRIPTION PLAN

A prescription vendor is an insurance company that manages your prescription plan. This is usually not the same company as your medical insurance. People frequently call their medical insurance company and take their frustration out on them, when they aren't even connected to the prescription vendor that can address the issue. As discussed in chapter 1, the different categories of insurance—medical, prescription, dental, and vision—are usually managed by different companies. Common prescription vendors are CVS Caremark, Express Scripts, and Optum Rx.

HEALTHCARE KNOWLEDGE: COPAY ASSISTANCE CARDS AND CASH-PRICE COUPONS

Not one person at the pharmacy has ever told me about copay cards or cash-price coupons, which can be used to lower your prescription costs. It is likely that nobody will tell you that there are copay cards or cash-price coupons to lower the price of your medication.

First, pharmacy staff are indisputably busy and don't want to do the work of entering in an additional four sets of numbers for those copay or cash-price coupons. Second, they may get reprimanded for unfavorably affecting the company's bottom line by going below the pharmacy's "cash price"; this could even put them at risk of termination or other punitive action. So pharmacy workers will tell you the cash price or the contracted cost of the medication, through your insurance, and that be that. They may let you become upset, then shift the blame onto your insurance company or doctor. They're not trying to wrong you, they're just providing you with the cash price or the insurance's contracted cost. It is up to you to actively find copay cards or cash-price coupons and request that they apply them, so that you receive the discount.

Here's what you need to know: There are copay assistance cards for almost all brand-name medications, and cash-price coupons for almost all generic medications. You have to meet certain qualifications, but they are relatively loose requirements. Unlike patient assistance programs, copay cards for brand-name medications don't have an income requirement. If you have commercial insurance through your employer or yourself, you usually meet the qualifications. You're ineligible for copay assistance cards if you have government funded insurance like Medicare, Medicaid, or Tricare.

Unfortunately, most medical providers won't offer to tell you about copay cards or cash-price coupons because they know you'll ask them to help you find and sign up for them, and they genuinely don't have the time. As a nurse practitioner in community medicine, in a clinic that served uninsured patients, I would frequently help many of my patients find and sign up for copay cards for each of their medications. I began doing this because many patients would come back for their three-month follow-up visit and tell me they never began the new medication because they couldn't afford it. Instead of calling the office to ask for assistance or looking into other options, they would go without these important medications.

Once I recognized this pattern, I began to help my patients find copay cards or cash-price coupons for the specific medications I was prescribing. This would take an excessive amount of time each day, so I can understand why most doctors don't offer this kind of assistance. This was awfully time consuming and I realized why medical providers I'd seen in the past, didn't communicate that there are copay cards and cash-price coupons, to help me afford the medications. However, there has to be a solution to the problem of unaffordable medications. I want to empower patients with this knowledge, so that they have the tools to access their medications through affordable pricing.

As an insurance customer care advocate, I've learned that most copay cards count toward your deductible. This makes sense, in my opinion, since the pharmaceutical company is literally paying your prescription copay when a copay card is used, and money is money, no matter where it comes from.

However, not all insurance companies accept these funds toward your deductible, so be sure to seek clarification on this matter with your insurance company.

However, if you use a cash-price coupon, such as GoodRx, it does not automatically count toward your deductible. You should submit the prescription and receipt to your prescription company's claims department to guarantee that the money you paid counts toward your deductible. Otherwise, that amount won't count toward your deductible or out-of-pocket balance.

RESPONSIBLE RESEARCH: TRY ALL OPTIONS AND ASK FOR ASSISTANCE

When you run into problems with a prescription, you should know who your prescription vendor is before you call the wrong number and cuss out the wrong person. In other words, make sure you're calling the prescription vendor to address any issues related to medications.

If you had a PA approval on a medication with one plan and then switched plans, you'll need to renew the PA for the Rx for the new plan. Whether it's a new plan in the same insurance company or an insurance plan change from one company to the next, begin the process to renew the PA as soon as possible.

Copay cards are available for almost every brand-name medication. It's your responsibility to find out the exact name, spelling, and indication (the condition being treated) of the medication in order to sign up for a copay card online. Some copay cards require you to sign up for them and then activate them. Be sure to look for this information to guarantee that the copay card works properly. Copay cards are for commercial insurance only—meaning for plans not funded by the government. Unfortunately, copay assistance cards cannot be used by anyone with government-funded primary-insurance such as Tricare, Medicare, or Medicaid.

In the rare case that you still cannot afford a medication with your insurance and a copay card, such as when you have a high deductible to meet or have government-funded insurance, ask your doctor for an alternative medication to use instead. A medication that has an exorbitant price may be a "higher tier" prescription, or it could even be a plan exclusion. A plan exclusion is a medication that an employer chose not to cover or that's excluded from the drug list that the employer chose based on the available packages and affordability.

When you cannot afford your medication and this is the only one that works, you should contact the drug manufacturer's patient assistance program. Almost every pharmaceutical company has a program that helps patients afford their medications. They mainly provide medication coverage for uninsured patients, but they will make exceptions if you speak to the right person and explain your circumstance. If a nurse advocate, a patient advocate, a medical provider, or you yourself write a letter explaining why that medication is needed and why you cannot afford it, the pharmaceutical company's patient assistance program will often be willing to work with you and provide some form of help.

Remember, copay assistance cards, cash-price coupons, and patient assistance programs are all excellent options when you can't afford the costs of your prescriptions.

CHAPTER 8

IMMUNIZATIONS

"Why was I just charged five hundred dollars for my shingles vaccine by my pharmacy? I was told it would be covered at 100 percent."

REALITY CHECK: AGE AND INDICATION

Immunizations prevent disease, and various vaccines are required at different ages and intervals throughout life. Most immunizations are covered at 100 percent under your preventative benefits. However, each immunization has its own specific age and indication requirements for coverage.

HEALTHCARE KNOWLEDGE: A MEDICAL BENEFIT, NOT A PHARMACY BENEFIT

Prescriptions aren't the only medical service provided by the pharmacy. Most immunizations can be given at in-network retail pharmacies, and are often covered very well as a preventative benefit. However, immunizations are a medical benefit, not a pharmacy benefit. Therefore, any time you request an immunization from your pharmacy, ensure that they run your medical insurance instead of your pharmacy or prescription insurance. This will prevent the frustration of being overcharged.

When possible, go to your local retail pharmacy for immunizations. There is no risk of being charged for an office-visit fee when you go to a retail pharmacy for vaccines. When you go to your doctor's office for immunizations, there is a risk you will have to pay for a nurse visit or office visit. This can come as quite a surprise when you're still in the process of meeting your deductible.

RESPONSIBLE RESEARCH: CHECK FOR AGE AND INDICATION REQUIREMENTS

Prior to getting an immunization, make sure that you meet the age and indication criteria for it. For example, one of the shingles vaccinations is usually covered as early as age fifty while the other one requires that you be at least sixty years old. The HPV vaccination is often covered from ages twelve to twenty-six years old in both. Pneumonia vaccinations are often covered at sixty years of age and older. These are just examples. Prior to receiving an immunization, call your insurance company to make sure it's covered.

CHAPTER 9

PREVENTIVE SERVICES

"Why did I receive a bill in the mail for my colonoscopy? It was a preventive screening that should've been covered at 100 percent!"

REALITY CHECK: NO SIGNS OR SYMPTOMS

I've received many a call from an upset patient who has gotten a bill for their colonoscopy, which they had believed would be covered 100 percent under their prevention benefits. This is a very confusing situation, and often there's no simple way to get it covered as a preventive service. A prevention-based screening screens for issues prior to any signs or symptoms of an illness. Prevention-based benefits include annual wellness exams, immunizations, mammograms, pap smears, colonoscopies, and a limited number of blood tests. Everything else is usually considered diagnostic in nature (diagnostic tests and procedures are ordered to determine the cause of a problem). The amount you are charged always goes back to how the doctor billed for the services he or she provided.

HEALTHCARE KNOWLEDGE: PREVENTIVE RULES, GUIDELINES, AND POLICIES

A patient will often go in for a screening colonoscopy, where the gastrointestinal specialist removes a precancerous polyp during the procedure, and end up with an unexpected bill. This occurs because the doctor will most likely submit coding for a colonoscopy that involves removal of a polyp. Upon receiving the doctor's invoice, the insurance company will run the claim according to the services listed in the billing codes. The doctor is not trying to wrong you, but is simply listing the services provided.

Unless a predetermination of benefits or prior authorization was submitted to the insurance company, the insurance company will have no idea that the procedure was supposed to be covered as a preventive service. This is why it's always a good idea to request that your doctor's office submit a predetermination of benefits *before* you go in for a procedure. With the predetermination of benefits, you can submit an appeal to the insurance company and fight the bill, stating that the service was supposed to be preventive and should be covered as so.

Another possible way you can contest an unanticipated bill like this, is to call your insurance company and ask if their preventive policy includes examples of preventive coverage along the lines of "a service is covered under the prevention-based benefit, when a diagnostic or therapeutic procedure occurs at the same time as the preventive procedure, as long as the procedure was scheduled as a preventive procedure or screening". You can attempt to have the claim reprocessed by talking to a supervisor, explaining that the procedure was preventive and mentioning the relevant language in the insurance's preventive rules. If they won't reprocess the bill, then you can initiate an appeal and involve your medical provider; request that the provider write a letter stating the procedure was scheduled as preventive because you've not had any signs, symptoms, or a history that would require a diagnostic procedure. Submit the appeal to the insurance company, firmly requesting that it be covered at 100 percent, consistent with your prevention-based benefits.

When filing an appeal it would be in your best interest to explain that your benefits or the company's preventive policy state something along the lines of "a service is covered under the prevention-based benefit, when a diagnostic or therapeutic procedure occurs at the same time as the preventive procedure, as long as the procedure was scheduled as a preventive procedure or screening" *and* that your doctor supports your claim that the procedure was planned as preventive. There is no guarantee that the insurance company will reprocess the claim or that your appeal will be approved, but it improves the chance of it being covered by the preventive benefit that you believe it should be covered under.

RESPONSIBLE RESEARCH: DON'T ASSUME YOUR PROVIDER KNOWS IT SHOULD BE PREVENTIVE

I once went in for a wellness exam and the wonderful physician assistant who regularly sees me, coded it as a condition management visit, instead of an annual wellness visit. She did this because, like most healthcare providers, she is very busy and frequently sees patients for disease management visits throughout the day. I knew it was an accident, but it was I who had to deal with the bill. I called the office and asked her to change it ,and then I asked my insurance company to reprocess the claim now that the coding was corrected. Everything ended up fine.

Embarrassingly enough, I've made this mistake myself, as a nurse practitioner, when seeing patients with commercial insurance. I was so used to seeing uninsured patients that I would forget to code the visit as a wellness exam because insurance was something I rarely dealt with. You can prevent this from happening to you by respectfully communicating with your medical provider. Prior to having a preventive wellness exam or screening procedure, tell your provider that you believe that this office visit or procedure is preventive in nature, and request that they bill it as such. Remember, your medical provider is thinking about your medical needs, not your coverages. Medical providers are not billing and coding experts; they do the best they can with what they know and the services they've delivered.

When you go to your primary care physician's office for an annual wellness exam, be very clear with the front-desk staff and your provider that this is a preventive visit. Make sure the front desk schedules it as a wellness physical exam and that the clinician knows to conduct a preventive visit instead of a disease management one. Just be aware that this visit won't address any signs or symptoms of any current medical problems.

CHAPTER 10

REFERRALS TO SPECIALISTS AND SURGEONS

"Would you trust this surgeon to operate on a close member of your family?"

REALITY CHECK: RESEARCH REFERRALS FOR YOURSELF

When a medical provider refers you to a specialist or a surgeon, be sure to look into the referred provider yourself. Most medical providers who make referrals, do so with the best interest of their patients, as their foremost concern; however, this is not always the case. Some physicians may actually refer patients to another physician to cultivate business relations or personal reasons. This can also occur when a physician is referring a patient to a specific facility for a diagnostic test or procedure.

Although, this is not always the case, I've seen numerous medical providers refer patients to their friends and those with whom they want to maintain working relationships, paying less consideration to patient-centered factors. This is more common than you might think, especially in the case of surgeon and facility referrals. To be clear, the point is to be aware of where a referral might be coming from and to do the necessary research before making a decision.

HEALTHCARE KNOWLEDGE: "BEST DOCTORS" LISTS

Several physicians I've worked with have been listed in regional magazines as among the area's "Best Doctors." Many of them, I believe, have deserved that status, due to their high quality of work and excellent patient outcomes. However, there have been other "Best Doctors" whom I would not personally recommend to family or friends, based on what I've observed of their work in the hospital. This is why I do not fully trust these listings. Additionally, colleagues have told me that such lists serve primarily as advertisements paid for by doctors' offices rather than as unbiased evaluations of medical care from patients.

If you read the details about the different lists available, you'll see that many of them are doctors nominated by other doctors, and few are nominated by patients they've treated. There are many high-quality medical providers available to you. I encourage you to do your own research, to take these published rankings with a grain of salt, and determine for yourself if a recommended specialist or surgeon is a good fit for your needs.

RESPONSIBLE RESEARCH: TALK TO OTHERS, DO ONLINE RESEARCH, AVOID BIASED REVIEWS

When you are referred to a specialist or a surgeon, do more than simply check whether the doctor is in or out of network. Researching your prospective provider can be as simple as asking another patient about them and as detailed as looking into their credentials.

One of the best ways to learn about a medical provider is to ask friends and family about their firsthand experiences with them. However, it's important to remember that someone else's experience with a particular provider will not necessarily reflect your own. Carefully consider what you are seeking in a physician for your particular set of needs.

At the very least, do a general online search. Search engines and social media will yield patient reviews, the provider's educational background, and miscellaneous details. Be wary of obviously biased reviews, positive or negative. As long as you use common sense and sound judgment, you can generally learn about a medical provider's overall attitude, credentials, and bedside manner in this way.

CHAPTER 11

SURGERY

"Why did I receive separate bills from the surgeon and anesthesiologist, if I already paid the hospital for the surgery?"

REALITY CHECK: THERE ARE MULTIPLE COSTS ASSOCIATED WITH SURGERY

A lot of patients assume that the hospital (or medical facility) fee is the only charge they will be responsible for when going in for a surgery, procedure, or emergency room visit. I have received many calls from upset patients, demanding to know why the doctor and anesthesiologist sent them bills in addition to the hospital bill they received.

Unfortunately, the fee paid to the medical facility does not include the cost of the doctor actually performing the surgery or the cost of anesthesia. Most surgeons and other physicians are contracted by a hospital to provide services to patients; they're not usually an employee of the hospital, so they must bill independently for their services.

Surgery involves many different benefit types, it is not a bundle deal. These categories often include anesthesia, surgical services, lab work, pathology, and the medical facility charges A medical facility may be a hospital, outpatient surgery center, diagnostic center, or other facility that performs medical procedures. The facility fee covers supplies, employees, and the physical space used at the hospital or outpatient surgery center. It often covers lab work as well; although it's rare, there are times when lab work and pathology are also billed independently of the hospital fee.

Therefore, be prepared to pay multiple types of medical fees for a surgery, diagnostic procedure, or emergency room visit. Note in advance the different fees involved and expect to receive separate bills for each service provided.

HEALTHCARE KNOWLEDGE: THE CUSTOMER CARE ADVOCATE, PROBABLY WON'T BE ABLE TO TELL YOU THE COSTS OF YOUR UPCOMING SURGERY, THERE IS A REASON.

The surgeon's office manager, or their surgery scheduler, should be able to list all of the estimated costs for your upcoming surgery. Each time I've had surgery, the office manager or surgery scheduler has been the one to provide me with this information.

Patients frequently call the insurance company asking for their out-of-pocket costs for an upcoming surgery. For a very limited number of procedures, your insurance company may be able to provide you with an estimate, but it is better equipped to provide you with estimated costs of labs and imaging. Due to the complexity of most surgical procedures, it may be impossible for the insurance company to provide you with cost estimates of your scheduled surgery.

Each medical provider, anesthesia group, and medical facility has a different contracted rate with your insurance company. The surgeon's office and medical facility should be able to provide you with details of expected out-of-pocket costs because they have contracted rates for the services they provide on file. Unfortunately, the customer care advocate or insurance company representative rarely has access to these rates, due to the vast number of providers, facilities, and procedures.

RESPONSIBLE RESEARCH: SEARCH FOR A FACILITY THAT CHARGES LESS

Surgeons often have "privileges" to work out of many different facilities. They may only work out of certain facilities on set days of the week. One of these facilities may be significantly more expensive than another—an especially important factor to consider if you've not yet met your in-network deductible or out-of-pocket maximum.

Ask the surgery scheduler for a list of facility prices for your surgery. Although you may have originally wanted to have surgery on a Friday, a large difference in cost may convince you to have surgery on another day at another facility with the same doctor.

When I was having a tonsillectomy, the surgery scheduler kept urging me to have it done at this one facility, but the price seemed very high, despite the fact that I had already met my deductible. This facility charged a lot more than the other facility that the ear, nose, and throat specialist worked out of, so I switched the day of the week I would have the surgery and saved over a thousand dollars.

Don't be afraid to ask the office manager or surgery scheduler about your facility options. At best, you will save yourself a considerable amount of money. At worst, you will learn that there is only one facility that has the equipment or level of care you need. For example, if you have multiple health conditions and have a higher risk of developing a postoperative issue, the surgeon may only be willing to operate on you at a level-one hospital that provides care to those with severe illnesses, which will likely charge more than a smaller hospital or surgery center.

CHAPTER 12

MATERNITY CARE

"I am pregnant, so all of my maternity care is covered at 100 percent, right? It's not a sickness or illness, after all".

REALITY CHECK: PREGNANCY IS CONSIDERED A MEDICAL CONDITION

Maternity services are usually covered at the same rate as all inpatient hospital stays and procedures. A lot of people believe that pregnancy care is covered at 100 percent because they do not view having a baby as an illness or medical condition. Unfortunately, health insurance views pregnancy as it does other medical conditions—offering similar coverage for hospital stays, doctor's fees, diagnostics, and lab work. Most breast pumps are covered at 100 percent, one per pregnancy, as long as you have a prescription and use an in-network medical equipment vendor.

Healthcare reform has improved coverages for women's healthcare in regard to pregnancy, contraception, and preventive services. If your medical plan follows healthcare reform, you may have expanded care services for women's health needs. This often includes improved coverage for women's preventive care, breast pumps, and lactation assistance.

HEALTHCARE KNOWLEDGE: ADDING YOUR NEWBORN TO YOUR INSURANCE PLAN

The human resources department is the one that manages your insurance premiums, updates your address on file, and can add someone to your plan. Once your baby is born, you must call your insurance's human resources department to have your baby added to the plan. Some plans allow as many as sixty days to add your newborn to the policy, while other plans only allow a maximum of four days. When calling your insurance company to find out about maternity or breast pump benefits, be sure to ask how long you have to add your newborn to the health insurance policy.

RESPONSIBLE RESEARCH: FINDING AN IN-NETWORK LACTATION CONSULTANT

Seeing an in-network lactation consultant can be a confusing process. Lactation consultants are not usually considered "billable providers" because they do not have a national provider number. For lactation consulting to be covered as in-network, your ob-gyn, pediatrician, birthing facility, and/or hospital must be in-network with your insurance plan; and the lactation consultant must bill under the name of the in-network provider or in-network facility. Contact your ob-gyn, pediatrician, birthing facility, or hospital to set up lactation consultant services. Many lactation consultants work in an in-network doctor's office where the service is billed under the provider or office name.

However, if the lactation consultant is an independent contractor or does not bill under the in-network provider or facility, then it won't be covered at the in-network rate, and may not be covered at all.

CHAPTER 13

EMERGENCY ROOMS V. URGENT CARE CLINICS

"Why is my bill so high? I thought I was seen by one of those urgent care clinics. I had no idea that building was an emergency room."

REALITY CHECK: FREE-STANDING ERS ARE NOT URGENT CARE CLINICS

It is important to remember that an emergency room is an emergency room, whether or not it is connected to a hospital. People habitually mistake free-standing ERs for urgent care clinics because they often resemble one another in outward appearance. Unfortunately, that's one of their only similarities.

Emergency rooms typically charge a much higher copay and tend to bill at a much higher rate than urgent care clinics. This dramatic difference between the two can come as a shock when you receive the bill in the mail, especially if you haven't met your deductible yet. Additionally, many free-standing emergency rooms are out-of-network, unless they're associated with an in-network hospital chain.

HEALTHCARE KNOWLEDGE: NON-EMERGENT VISITS TO AN ER MAY BE DENIED

I've seen claims denied because a patient was seen at an emergency room for a non-emergent disorder. Yes, they wanted to receive immediate medical care for a highly concerning problem, but the claim was denied because they did not technically have an *emergent* issue. An emergent condition is one that requires immediate life-sustaining intervention to prevent loss of life, limb, or vision. Unless you truly have an emergent problem, it's in your best interest to be seen by a primary care provider or an urgent care clinic.

There may be a time when you or a loved one are experiencing exacerbated symptoms of your condition and it seems like it might be an emergency.

I've received many calls from individuals who were genuinely concerned about safety but were on the fence about whether they or a loved one were experiencing an emergency or not, and the only facility open at the time was an emergency room. If you are concerned for yourself or a loved one due to certain signs and symptoms, it is always better to be safe than sorry. If you think it might be an emergency, please call 911 or go to the nearest ER.

If your claim is denied because you were seen at an emergency room for what is later considered a non-emergent condition, you have the right to appeal. It's worth the effort to appeal the denied claim if an emergency room was the only medical facility open at the time that you or a someone you know were experiencing intense symptoms—especially if you thought it may have been an emergent health condition that could not wait for an urgent care clinic to open the next morning. Explain to the insurance company the severity of the symptoms and make clear that there were no other options at the time. The insurance company will only receive the billing and diagnosis codes received by the medical provider, so this additional information must come from you.

It is up to you to appeal a denied claim and plead your case. There is no guarantee this will result in victory, but doing nothing guarantees defeat. Advocate for yourself and see if you can get the decision reversed.

RESPONSIBLE RESEARCH

Check your benefits in advance to determine if non-emergent conditions will be covered when seen at an emergency room, for situations like the one outlined above.

If you're ill and need medical attention, but it is not an emergency, first call your primary care provider to check their availability. If your primary care provider is unavailable, call your insurance company to find a list of urgent care clinics that are in-network. This can save you time and money.

If you're experiencing an emergency—in other words, if there is reasonable concern for loss of life, limb, or vision—call 911 or go to the nearest emergency room. In the event of an emergency, the only thing that matters is safety, and an ER's network status should not matter. You can always contact insurance customer after the fact and plead your case.

CHAPTER 14

INTELLECTUAL AND DEVELOPMENTAL DELAYS

"My child is struggling in school and I am concerned that he has a developmental delay. How do I get him help?"

REALITY CHECK: A CONFUSING AND SENSITIVE MEDICAL ISSUE

It can be difficult to know what path to take when you're concerned about your child having a learning disability or cognitive delay. Knowing how or where to begin the assessment process is often confusing and intimidating to a parent trying to address this type of sensitive medical issue. I recently helped a friend in this situation, and it took some trial and effort, but I was able to discover a reasonable course of action that may benefit others in similar circumstances. Fortunately, though also confusingly, there are multiple ways to address your child's needs.

HEALTHCARE KNOWLEDGE: TACKLE THE PROBLEM THROUGH MEDICAL AND PSYCHOLOGICAL ASSESSMENT

First, I recommend that you have your child evaluated by his or her pediatrician. The pediatrician will be able to tell you whether they believe there's cause for concern. If so, the doctor can advise you on next steps to take and other resources. If your child's pediatrician does not believe that the issue is necessarily cognitive, you will want to rule out other underlying physical or psychological issues, by seeing specialists.

The pediatrician can direct you to other clinicians who can further assess your child, such as an ophthalmologist to address a vision impairment, an audiologist to address a hearing impairment, or a neurologist to address a neurological disorder. These providers can help to identify or rule out an underlying medical cause. Your pediatrician may also refer your child to a developmental pediatrician, psychiatrist, or a pediatric psychologist, to rule out an underlying mental health issue. Your insurance company's customer service department can help you find in-network clinicians in all of these areas.

RESPONSIBLE RESEARCH: FIND AN EDUCATIONAL DIAGNOSTICIAN

Meanwhile, in addition to seeking medical expertise, one of the most important things you can do is to request that your child's school have an educational diagnostician evaluate him or her for learning disabilities. Some schools require a handwritten request. If your child attends public school, request that the school district's diagnostician assess your child for limitations in intellectual functioning. Most public school districts have educational diagnosticians who test students for learning impairments. In the event that your public school district doesn't have a diagnostician, ask the principal to see if a neighboring district can provide assistance. In my friend's case, it was the public school's diagnostician who identified the problem; the pediatrician ruled out medical causes. The child was placed in a more appropriate learning environment and is now excelling.

CHAPTER 15

CALLING THE INSURANCE COMPANY

"You denied my life-sustaining medication and you won't cover my procedure! What is the point of paying my premiums?"

REALITY CHECK: CUSTOMER SERVICE IS NOT THE ENEMY

Patients call their insurance companies every day, taking their anger out on customer service representatives, who are the ones who want to help and have nothing to do with the problem. So when you call customer service with a complaint, realize that the person who answers the phone will have no clue what has occurred on your end until they open several screens in your account. The nicer you are to the customer service rep, the more they'll want to help and the more information they'll provide to help relieve the problem.

Remember, it's frequently your employer who changed what was covered or not, not the insurance. The insurance company is only working off what they were told to include in the plan. Although it's rare, the insurance company could have changed details in the plan, but it's usually the employer who selects coverages for their employees' health insurance package.

HEALTHCARE KNOWLEDGE: WHEN YOU ARE GIVEN WRONG INFORMATION

If an employee of the insurance company has made a mistake and given you incorrect information about coverage, the insurance company will most likely honor it and cover any related costs. However, the patient must bring it to the attention of the billing department or a supervisor. They will not offer to correct this issue, you'll have to firmly request that they do.

For example, if someone at the insurance company told you that a medical provider or facility was in-network, but they weren't, most insurance companies will cover the costs at the in-network rate. If you receive a large bill because you were given incorrect information, call the insurance company and request to speak to a supervisor about the problem. Most, if not all, calls are recorded. Ask the supervisor to review both the documentation and the voice recording of the call, from the date you were told the incorrect information; so that they can verify your story. Then ask the supervisor to reprocess the claims at the promised in-network benefit.

There is no guarantee that the insurance company will reprocess your claim or that your appeal will be approved, but it improves the chances of it being covered by the benefit you believed it would be covered under.

RESPONSIBLE RESEARCH: BE PREPARED TO COMMUNICATE CLEARLY

When calling your insurance company, be prepared to state the problem clearly and let them know the medication is important to your health, and they will work hard to fix the issue. Telling the customer service agent a long story about why you need the medication, saying you've been taking it for over twenty years, and offering your opinion on why this should be approved won't help anything—especially if you do so in an aggressive or condescending tone. If additional documentation, a letter of medical necessity, a peer-to-peer call, or other PA information is required by the clinical services department from your doctor, tell your doctor. Here are some examples of what to tell your doctor to include in a PA request:

- You've tried everything else but nothing else works.
- You've been on this medication for twenty years.
- You've had certain negative reactions to lower-cost alternatives.

Your doctor can include those details in the medical necessity report they send to the clinical services department to request prescription approval.

CONCLUSION

Like any complex system run by human beings, the healthcare system is susceptible to miscommunication and errors. However, its main purpose is to aid you, the patient, when you need it. If you run into problems with your healthcare coverage, it's vitally important that you remember to persevere and utilize various resources available to assist you.

With the information I've provided in this book, I hope you will now have the courage and wherewithal to stand up and advocate for yourself whenever you hit a roadblock. Managing your healthcare can be tedious and frustrating, but making the effort to understand how it works, familiarize yourself with the details of your health plan, and communicate clearly with each party involved will pay off hugely in the end—in the form of better care and significantly lower bills.

Each and every time you encounter an issue, reach out to someone for assistance so that the problem can be resolved. Keep this book handy and refer back to it often—whenever you need a bit of encouragement and advice. Calm perseverance is key when searching for a solution to a healthcare service mix-up. As someone who has been there, on both ends of the customer service line, I wish you the very best as you continue, newly empowered, on your healthcare journey!

ACKNOWLEDGMENTS

I would also like to thank all of my family, friends, patients, members, and clients whom I've helped over the years. You have inspired me to share my experiences and unique perspective; my hope in sharing these experiences, is to provide relief, and help as many people as I possibly can.

HEALTHCARE NAVIGATION CHECKLIST

1. Please, actively read the benefit package given to you every year by your employer or, for an individual plan, sent to you directly after open enrollment. Be sure to read it not only the first year of employment, but also each subsequent year when you renew your insurance. Be aware of your plan details, coverages, benefits, deductibles, out-of-pocket maximums, copays, and co-insurance responsibilities. This and all other details can be found in your benefit package.

2. Request that the doctor's office do a predetermination (pre-D) of benefits before any office visit, lab work, diagnostic test, high-tier medication, treatment, procedure, or surgery.

3. If a medical service requires prior authorization (PA), request your doctor's office submit the PA at least two weeks in advance. PAs may be required for tests, treatments, medications, procedures, or surgeries.

4. Verify with your insurance's customer service department that a medical provider is in-network prior to seeing them in their office. Also, check to make sure that the address you will be going to is in-network. For example, a doctor might work out of three office locations while only two of them could be in-network for you.

5. Verify that any and all facilities are in-network prior to physically going to the facility and receiving services. These facilities include laboratories, imaging centers,

doctor's offices, satellite office locations, surgery centers, general hospitals, emergency rooms, convenience care clinics, urgent care clinics, pharmacies, and any other form of medical building that you may need to go to for medical services.

6. Tell each of your doctors which lab facility is in-network for you, so they can factor this in when completing an order form. This will increase the likelihood that they will send you to an in-network lab facility for blood work. However, don't assume that the referred lab is in-network; always double-check before having your blood drawn.

7. Shop for the best price when your doctor orders diagnostic or imaging tests. This can be done through your insurance's cost estimation tool in your patient portal online or by calling your insurance agency's customer service department.

8. Search, register, and activate copay assistance cards for all brand-name medications. When your prescriptions costs are still too high, take advantage of patient assistance programs.

9. Search for cash-price coupons to lower the costs of generic medications when you cannot afford them through insurance.

10. Request that your doctor renew your medication's prior authorization a month before its expiration date to avoid any gaps in coverage. Remember that PAs for medication are only good for a twelve-month period, so initiate renewal in advance.

FREQUENTLY ASKED QUESTIONS: MISCELLANEOUS

"I HAVE CANCER, SO EVERYTHING IS COVERED AT 100 PERCENT, RIGHT?"

Most patients believe that cancer, dialysis, and transplant services are covered at 100 percent. Unfortunately, they're not. Cancer, dialysis, and transplant services are usually covered at the same rate as all other treatments and procedures.

"MY HUSBAND IS ON THE LIVER TRANSPLANT LIST, SO HIS AMBULANCE RIDES ARE COVERED 100 PERCENT AS AN EMERGENCY, CORRECT?"

What you believe to be an emergency or an urgent matter may not match what the doctor or insurance company defines as urgent. For a condition to qualify as an emergency, it must require immediate life-sustaining intervention to prevent loss of life, limb, or vision. This is the common knowledge term used to describe and define an emergency.

If you're unsure what to do, you can always call your insurance's nurse-line for advice on the best course of action. The answering nurse can let you know whether it makes sense to stay home and wait to see the doctor or to go to the ER right way. You can typically find the nurse-line number on the back of your insurance card.

"I THOUGHT MY BIRTH CONTROL WAS COVERED AT 100 PERCENT. WHY AM I BEING CHARGED FOR IT?"

Through healthcare reform, most types of birth control are covered at 100% of costs, when they are prescribed for the sole purpose of contraception. If the birth control type medication is prescribed for a reason other than contraception, such as irregular menstrual periods, then it becomes subject to the deductible and coverage resorts back to the plan's prescription benefits.

"I AM RESIGNING FROM MY JOB AND I WILL BE SELF-EMPLOYED SOON. I WILL LOSE COVERAGE WITH YOUR INSURANCE COMPANY. IN ORDER TO OBTAIN COVERAGE THROUGH MY SPOUSE'S INSURANCE COMPANY, I NEED PROOF THAT I DON'T HAVE INSURANCE COVERAGE. WHY CAN'T YOU SEND ME THE LETTER TODAY?"

A letter showing proof that a person has lost insurance coverage, cannot be generated until the insurance plan has formally ended. Once your insurance coverage has terminated, call the insurance company to request the letter. They are often called "proof of lost coverage letters". They cannot generate a letter that shows when your coverage is suspected to end.

"WHY WAS MY BABY NOT AUTOMATICALLY ADDED TO MY INSURANCE POLICY WHEN HE WAS BORN?"

Once your baby is born, you must call the subscriber's human resources department to have your baby added to the plan. Some plans allow as many as sixty days to add your newborn to the policy, while other plans only allow a maximum of four or five days to add the baby to the plan.

"WHY DOES ONE COMPANY COST MORE THAN THE OTHER COMPANY FOR THE SAME EXACT MEDICAL PRODUCT? SHOULDN'T IT ALL BE THE SAME SINCE THEY BOTH ACCEPT MY INSURANCE?"

Each in-network provider, whether it be a medical provider or a facility, has contracted rates with your insurance company. In-network providers can offer the same service, or the same piece of durable medical equipment, at different prices. This is because one company negotiated a better contracted rate with your insurance company, which is why they're able to offer the same product at a lower price than the other company, under your benefits. The contracted rate for services and supplies can vary due to multiple factors.

"I'LL BE OUT OF STATE FOR THE NEXT FEW WEEKS. CAN I GET A VACATION OVERRIDE FOR MY MEDICAL SUPPLIES, LIKE I HAVE DONE FOR MY MEDICATIONS IN THE PAST?"

Unlike prescription medications, there are usually no sort of vacation override for medical equipment supplies. Your doctor's office or medical supply company can submit a prior authorization for a limit increase, but this may take up to two weeks;

meaning that you may already be on vacation by the time a decision is reached.

The best thing to do is call the durable medical equipment company and ask them to deliver the supplies to your out-of-state vacation address when the new shipment is available. This only works if you're vacationing within the country; if you are out of the country, it may be best to have it delivered to a friend or family member and have them ship it to your international destination. Medical supply company's don't often deliver internationally but they may for an additional fee; each company varies.

"ONCE I MEET MY IN-NETWORK DEDUCTIBLE, EVERYTHING IS COVERED AT 100 PERCENT, CORRECT?"

No, you are responsible for paying for all out-of-pocket costs, until you meet your in-network deductible. Benefits kick-in once your in-network deductible is satisfied. Your plan begins to pay a portion of your covered health services once you've met your deductible. Out-of-network deductible and coverages are separate from in-network deductible and coverages.

"I HAVE MEDICAL COVERAGE THROUGH TWO DIFFERENT INSURANCE COMPANIES. THEY'LL BOTH COVER THE TOTAL BILL, SO I WON'T HAVE TO PAY ANYTHING OUT OF POCKET, CORRECT?"

Unfortunately, most insurance plans have a stipulation that doesn't allow for double coverage of the same medical service. This means that the secondary insurance doesn't often cover the remaining out-of-pocket costs. The only time a secondary insurance company will pay for anything, is if their coverage for that benefit covered a larger percentage of the costs, than the primary insurance benefits covered. Most secondary insurance plans will only pay as much as they would pay, if they were the patient's only insurance company; the secondary insurance company determines the amount they will cover, as if the primary insurance company wasn't involved.

For example, if you have a procedure done and your primary insurance company covers the procedure at 80 percent and your secondary insurance company covers the procedure at 80 percent, then you're still responsible for the remaining 20 percent. The secondary insurance company won't cover the remaining bill; they'll only cover what they would have, as if they were the only insurance company. Since your primary insurance company already covered 80 percent, then they won't pay anything additional because all they would consider covering was the same 80 percent that has already been covered by the primary insurance.

To illustrate this further, if you have a procedure done and your primary insurance company covers the procedure at 70 percent and your secondary insurance company covers the procedure at 90 percent, then you're only responsible for the remaining 10 percent. The secondary insurance company would cover 20 percent of the total bill because their benefit percentage was higher than the primary insurance benefit. The primary insurance company covered the initial 70 percent of the cost; while the secondary covered 20 percent, for a total of 90 percent, because they would've covered 90 percent of the procedure if they were the only insurance company.

GLOSSARY

Calendar Year Plan: A health insurance plan that follows the calendar year, beginning on January 1 and ending on December 31 of the same year.

Cash-Price Coupon: A discount on the pharmacy's retail price of the medication, the price you would pay without using health insurance.

Claims or Billing Representative: An employee of the insurance company who addresses financial issues or researches financial details related to services that have already occurred.

Co-Insurance: Insurance coverage for a portion of your medical expenses. For example, some plans cover 70 percent of medical expenses while you cover 30 percent, whereas other plans cover 90 percent of medical expenses while you cover 10 percent of the costs.

Commercial Insurance: Insurance accessed through an individual or employment plan. No form of government-funded insurance is commercial insurance.

Convenience Care Clinic: A small clinic that can see you for basic preventive care, such as physical exam or immunizations. It can also treat mild illnesses. This type of clinic supplements the care offered by most primary care providers without the long wait time for an appointment. A convenience care clinic does not take the place of a primary care provider, an urgent care clinic, or an emergency room; rather, it is a place of service that's intended to decrease the number of people waiting in an urgent care clinic or emergency room for minor issues.

Copay: A set fee that a health insurer requires a patient to pay for certain services covered by the plan. Copays can be for doctor's office visits, prescriptions, and inpatient hospital stays. Copays do not usually go toward your deductible, and your deductible is not usually a factor when a copay covers the set benefit.

Copay Card: Copay cards lower the out-of-pocket or copay costs of brand-name medications for patients with commercial insurance plans. Copay cards don't usually lower the cost of medications if you have Medicare, Medicaid, or Tricare.

Current Procedural Terminology (CPT) Codes: CPT codes are detailed numbers used for the billing of medical services.

Deductible: The amount you pay out of pocket for medical care and prescriptions, at the contracted rate for in-network providers and facilities. Once you reach the deductible, the health insurance coverages begin. This usually comes in the form of co-insurance.

Diagnostics: Lab work, imaging, or other tests that aid in diagnosis of a disorder or illness.

Emergency: A medical emergency occurs when there is immediate or present risk of loss of life, limb, and/or vision.

Hospitalist: A medical provider, usually a physician, contracted by a hospital to care for inpatients.

Imaging: An X-ray, ultrasound, CT scan, MRI, or other medical imaging.

In-Network: Describes a medical provider or facility that has contracted with your health insurance company to accept certain negotiated rates.

Inpatient: A patient who stays in a medical facility for more than twenty-four hours.

Medical Provider: A doctor, physician, physician assistant, nurse practitioner, chiropractor, physical therapist, or other billable provider.

Nurse Practitioner: A registered nurse with advanced training who can assess, diagnose, and treat patients. A nurse practitioner has more autonomy than a registered nurse but usually still works under a delegating physician, and does not do surgical procedures on their own.

Out-of-Network (OON): Describes a medical provider or facility that does not have a contract with your health insurance company.

Outpatient: A patient who stays in a medical facility for less than twenty-four hours.

Out-of-Pocket Maximum: The maximum amount of money you will spend toward medical services for the remainder of the plan year. Most, but not all, plans allow copays to go toward the out-of-pocket maximum.

Patient Advocate: Someone who acts in the best interest of the patient. For example, a patient advocate could call on the patient's behalf to get an issue resolved, provide resources, or assist the patient with any number of tasks.

Physician Assistant: A medical provider much like a nurse practitioner who can assess, diagnose, and treat patients. A physician assistant has more autonomy than a registered nurse but usually works under a delegating physician, and does not do surgical procedures on their own.

Plan Exclusion: A medical service, procedure, medication, or piece of equipment not covered by the insurance.

Policy Year Plan: A health insurance plan that follows a twelve-month period that can start at any point in the calendar year, determined by the employer.

Pre-Approval: The terms "pre-approval" and "prior authorization" are often used interchangeably. The insurance must verify that a medication, surgery, or other medical service is medically safe and necessary in accordance with current medical guidelines.

Predetermination of Benefits: A request for services that your doctor submits to your insurance company to determine if it will be covered and how much your responsibility will be. This is to see if things will be covered, in general—not like a prior authorization, where the service requested is checked against medical guidelines for the condition to determine if it is safe, efficient, and medically necessary.

Prior Authorization: The terms "pre-approval" and "prior authorization" are often used interchangeably. The insurance must verify that a medication, surgery, or other medical service is medically safe and necessary in accordance with current medical guidelines.

Specialist: Any doctor, physician, nurse practitioner, or physician assistant who specializes in a certain field of medicine.

Surgeon: A doctor or physician who has received extensive education and training in a specialized field of medicine that involves surgical correction of the disorder.

Urgent Care Clinic: A medical clinic that cares for patients with a sickness, minor injury, and other urgent care needs, including allergic reactions and asthma attacks. These clinics are usually open on weekends and have extended hours during weekdays.

Vendor: A company that manages a certain area of your medical care—such as medical, prescription, dental, vision, and/or medical equipment—independent of the insurance company.

Made in the USA
Middletown, DE
05 November 2026

36544880R10068